CHROMOTHERAPY

A Guided Exploration Of Wellness Through The Rainbow Spectrum: Discover The Healing Power Of Colors And Transform Your Life

Nuel Nenji

Contents

Introductory

One form of complementary medicine that makes use of color to improve health is chromotherapy, sometimes called color therapy. The basic premise of chromotherapy is that different hues elicit different physiological and psychological reactions in humans. Those who believe in the curative power of color theory put up the idea of chromotherapy.

Some commonly held beliefs about the effects of different colors in chromotherapy are as follows:

• The color red is commonly linked to vitality, enthusiasm, and heightened blood flow. People feel it gives them more energy and bravery.

• The color orange is associated with a sense of harmony, vitality, and originality. It brings feelings of happiness and comfort.

• The color yellow is often linked to positivity, optimism, and intelligence. It is said that the color yellow might help one concentrate and communicate better.

• Harmony, balance, and healing are often associated with the color green. It is thought to be a soothing color that helps alleviate tension and unwind.

• The relaxing and soothing benefits of the color blue are well-known. Peace, understanding, and lucidity are some of its cherished qualities.

• Indigo: A stone said to heighten clairvoyance and enlightenment. It is thought to bring about states of profound meditation and contemplation.

• Spirituality, intuition, and tranquility of spirit are often linked with the violet and purple color palette. Its balancing and relaxing effects on the mind and body are widely thought to be true.

Some methods of chromotherapy include exposing the patient to colored lights, donning colored apparel, working with colored fabrics, or encircling oneself with certain hues in one's surroundings.

The scientific evidence for the efficacy of chromotherapy is minimal, however some people find it helpful for relaxation and stress reduction.

Individuals should go into chromotherapy with an open mind and sensitivity to their own preferences and sensitivities, as is the case with many alternative therapies, because its effects might differ from person to person. Seek the advice of a trained medical expert before deciding to undergo chromotherapy for any health-related reasons.

CHAPTER ONE
Evidence-Based Practices

Chromatotherapy has a weak scientific foundation, despite the fact that light and color can influence people's physiology and psychology. Rather than being a generally recognized medical profession, the area is sometimes seen as a form of alternative or supplementary medicine. Presented below are a few considerations:

• Colors have the power to affect our emotions and how we perceive the world around us. Certain colors may have a particular effect on people's emotions. This branch of psychology is called color psychology, and it has been around for a long time.

• Seasonal affective disorder (SAD) is one medical illness that has responded to light therapy, which involves exposure to light in all its color spectrums.

In light therapy, a bright light, similar to that of the sun, is used to alleviate some symptoms. Nevertheless, the color of the light is less important than its strength and wavelength.

• A person's sleep-wake cycles and general health are influenced by their circadian rhythms, which are regulated by light exposure, particularly natural sunlight. These rhythms can be affected by changes in color temperature of light, but what matters most are changes in overall brightness and the timing of light exposure.

• Although there is some study on the physiological and psychological effects of light and color, the particular assertions put out by chromotherapy practitioners sometimes do not have strong scientific backing.

More study is required to establish conclusive relationships between specific colors and treatment effects, as studies in this area are typically modest in scope.

It's important to keep an open mind when using chromotherapy and to remember that people have different reactions to different colors. One person's stimulating or relaxing experience may have the opposite impact on another.

Another factor that could influence the claimed effectiveness of chromotherapy is the placebo effect, which occurs when a person feels better because they believe in the treatment.

Talking to a doctor is a good idea before trying chromotherapy or any alternative treatment. In order to make sure that the strategy is in line with general health and wellness, they might give advice based on practices supported by evidence.

Choosing And Applying Colors

Color selection and application are crucial components of chromotherapy. Some broad principles for the possible selection and application of colors in chromotherapy are as follows:

1. Exploring the Relationships Between Colors:

- It is thought that certain hues evoke particular feelings, levels of energy, and physiological reactions.

- As an example, colors that are warm, like red and orange, are commonly linked to excitement and vitality, whereas colors that are cold, like green and blue, are linked to serenity and rest.

2. My Own Choices:

- Color sensitivity and the efficacy of chromotherapy are both affected by individual taste.
- Choosing colors for treatment requires careful consideration of each person's preferences.

3. Feelings and Situation:

- When choosing colors for chromotherapy, practitioners may rely on their intuition and take into account the unique circumstances of each patient's demands.

- A person looking to alleviate stress, for instance, could be shown soothing hues like green or blue.

4. Color Schemes for Unique Occurrences:

- Certain situations may call for the use of particular colors, according to some practitioners. The color yellow, for instance, could be suggested as a means to sharpen one's concentration and mental agility.

5. Application Methods:

- There are several methods to use chromotherapy, such as exposing oneself to colored lights, donning colored apparel, working with colored fibers, or encircling oneself with particular colors in one's surroundings.

- Certain uses call for the employment of color filters, colored lenses, or specially constructed light fixtures to produce a desired hue.

6. Time and Stress Level:

- Chromotherapy can be influenced by the length and strength of exposure to a specific color.

- To help you relax, it may be suggested to expose yourself to calming colors for a longer period of time, while to stimulate you, it may be suggested to expose yourself to stimulating colors for a shorter period of time.

7. Palette Harmony:

- To get a well-rounded look, some experts suggest using many hues.

- The desired outcome and specific aims of the therapy session may dictate the use of colors and their combinations.

8. Discussions with Medical Professionals:

- People who are curious about chromotherapy can seek advice from seasoned professionals who, after evaluating their requirements, will be able to suggest color applications tailored to their unique preferences.

It should be mentioned that although chromotherapy is utilized by some as an auxiliary method of health, there is little data to back its effectiveness.

It is important for people to talk to their doctors before trying chromotherapy or any alternative treatment, and to keep an open mind because everyone reacts differently.

CHAPTER TWO
Methods And Equipment For Chromotherapy

Chromatotherapy is the practice of using color for medicinal purposes using a variety of instruments and methods.

Proponents of chromotherapy employ these technologies to create environments or experiences based on color associations, even though the scientific basis is still under question. Some typical chromotherapy tools and procedures are as follows.

1. Various Hues:

- In chromotherapy, specialized light bulbs or fixtures are used to produce specific hues.

- One way to generate a colored atmosphere is by directing lights onto the body or into a room.

2. Color Adjustments:

- It is possible to create colored light by placing colored filters or lenses over light sources.

- Windows, lamps, and other light-emitting devices can all benefit from these filters.

3. Wearing Clothes of Different Colors:

- Some practitioners suggest that you wear specific colors or use specific textiles to boost your energy or mood.
- During therapy sessions, you can wear colorful clothes, drapes, or blankets.

4. Multi-Color Soak:

- As a form of chromotherapy, some individuals choose to soak in water that is lit by different colored lights.
- Some people think it can affect the body's energy levels

since the water absorbs the hue.

5. A Guide to Colour Meditation:

- As a component of chromotherapy, one may engage in meditation sessions with the intention of seeing or surrounding oneself with certain hues.
- People might be led to visualize a specific hue to help them rest or energize themselves.

6. Visualizing Colors:

- To accomplish an impact through visualization, one

must mentally fixate on a particular color.

- You can do this on your own or with the help of a professional.

7. Dissolving Dye:

- Some chromotherapy techniques include breathing exercises where the patient inhales and exhales specific hues.

- The premise is that the selected color's medicinal qualities are inhaled through the breath.

8. Crystals and Gemstones:

- Gemstones or crystals linked to particular colors are used in several chromotherapy procedures.
- The stones can be scattered around or applied directly to the skin.

9. Visual Aids for Color Therapy:

- Some practitioners employ colored lenses or spectacles that block off specific wavelengths.
- People put on these spectacles to feel the impact of certain hues.

10. Ambients that Alter Color:

- Chromotherapy is carried out in controlled surroundings with the ability to dynamically modify the illumination color.

- Projections or LED lights that change colors could be a part of these settings.

11. Procedure for administering dye:

- This method makes use of a tiny pen-like device to apply colored light to specific acupuncture sites on the skin.

- It is said by practitioners to promote energy flow and body equilibrium.

Because its efficacy is subjective and may differ among individuals, chromotherapy should be approached with skepticism. Furthermore, before adding chromotherapy to one's wellness routine, especially when coping with particular health issues, one should speak with healthcare providers.

Traditional Medical Chromatography

In conventional medical systems like Western medicine, Ayurveda, and Traditional Chinese Medicine (TCM), chromotherapy does not have the same level of recognition or acceptance as it does today.

These ancient medical systems have their own theories and procedures established in centuries of observation, experimentation, and cultural context.

In contrast, chromotherapy may not adhere to the tenets of conventional medicine since it is widely thought of as a supplemental or alternative treatment.

In a nutshell, chromotherapy is related to the following conventional medical practices:

1. Conventional Western Medicine:

- Practices and therapies in Western medicine are usually based on evidence.

- In Western medicine, chromotherapy—which centers on the therapeutic use of colors—is not widely practiced.

- Although certain diseases can be treated with light therapy, such SAD, the focus is on the wavelength and intensity of the light rather than certain hues.

2. Ayurveda practices:

- Finding a harmonious equilibrium among the three doshas—Vata, Pitta, and Kapha—is seen as vital to good health according to Ayurveda, India's traditional medical system.

- Ayurveda does make use of color in certain ways, but not

in the same way that chromotherapy does. Diet, lifestyle, and herbal medicines are all part of a more holistic approach to achieving balance, with colors representing the doshas.

3. Chinese medicine with a traditional focus:

- TCM centers on the idea of harmonizing the Qi (life force energy) and Chi (energetic chi) within the body.

- Although traditional Chinese medicine (TCM) acknowledges that environmental influences, such as colors, can impact health, it is not common practice in TCM to use specific colors for therapeutic purposes, like chromotherapy.

It's important to remember that traditional medical systems do acknowledge the impact of environmental influences, like colors, on health, even though chromotherapy isn't always central to them.

For example, traditional traditions like feng shui in Chinese culture consider the placement of things and colors in the environment to encourage harmony and balance.

Anyone thinking about trying chromotherapy or any other complementary or alternative medicine approach should talk to their doctor first to make sure it will help them achieve their health and wellness objectives.

CHAPTER THREE
Contemporary Use Cases

Despite chromotherapy's lack of support from conventional medical institutions, it continues to find use in complementary and alternative medicine. Several modern applications of chromotherapy include the following:

1. Health Clubs and Spas:

- Chromatin therapy is offered by some health clubs and spas. Colored lights can be used in saunas, baths, or relaxation rooms to create diverse atmospheres that are claimed to promote balance and relaxation.

2. Treatment of Mood Disorders with Light:

- Some forms of depression and Seasonal Affective Disorder (SAD) are treated using light therapy, which is also frequently referred to as chromotherapy.

- To mimic the effects of natural sunshine, light boxes are used that emit certain wavelengths of light instead of specific colors.

3. **Healthcare and Hospital Settings:**

- Using colored lighting can occasionally be employed in healthcare settings to establish a relaxing ambiance. In order to help patients rest, several facilities use calming colors like blue or green light in patient rooms.

4. **Changing Light Emitting Diodes:**

- To set the ambiance in their houses, some people use color-changing LED lights that can be controlled to change colors.

- Users of smart lighting systems can adjust the light's color temperature and brightness with the use of voice commands or mobile applications.

5. Creating a Beautiful Home:

- Designers of interior spaces often take into account the emotional and mental impacts of color schemes. For instance, bedrooms may be decorated with soothing colors, while places intended for socializing can be adorned with lively hues.

6.   Technology and its applications:

- The goal of certain apps and devices is to help you get a better night's sleep by adjusting the screen colors depending on the time of day. One such feature is the ability to limit exposure to blue light in the evening.

7. Technological Garments:

- Some eyeglasses and other wearables use light-emitting technology to supposedly provide chromotherapy by exposing the user to certain hues.

8. Wellness Routines:

- Instructors of mind-body disciplines, such as yoga and meditation, may direct students' attention to particular energy centers, or chakras, through the use of color visualizations.

Since there is no evidence that chromotherapy is effective as a treatment, it is crucial to approach these applications with skepticism. While it's true that some people find that certain colors help them relax or feel better, everyone reacts differently.

Seek the advice of medical experts before deciding to undergo chromotherapy, especially if you are coping with a serious medical issue.

A Healing Light's Potential

Light is fundamental to all forms of life on Earth and is involved in many important mental and physiological functions.

Light treatment for particular ailments is one example of a well-established method that makes use of light's therapeutic properties;

nevertheless, there are other, more speculative or alternative ideas, such as chromotherapy, that require further investigation.

The healing powers of light are recognized in the following ways:

1. Producing Vitamin D:

- Vitamin D can be naturally obtained from being exposed to sunlight. Essential for strong bones, healthy immune systems, and general health, vitamin D is produced by the skin when exposed to the sun's ultraviolet B (UVB) rays.

2. Regular Sleep Patterns:

- The body's internal clock, which controls when we sleep and when we get up, is regulated by exposure to natural light, particularly first thing in the morning.
- You can enhance your mood, vigilance, and quality of sleep by exposing yourself to light first thing in the morning.

3. A Treatment for Seasonal Affective Disorder (SAD) Through Light:

- Light therapy has a long history of success in treating

seasonal affective disorder, a form of seasonal depression that tends to hit during the winter months when sunshine exposure is at its lowest.

- To help with seasonal affective disorder (SAD), light boxes create a bright light that looks like sunlight.

4. Healing of Wounds:

- Researchers have looked at the possibility that specific light wavelengths, especially those in the red and near-infrared ranges, can aid in the healing of wounds and the repair of damaged tissues.

5. Skin Conditions Treated by Phototherapy:

- Dermatologists employ light therapy to alleviate symptoms of psoriasis and vitiligo, among others. In certain cases, controlled exposure to ultraviolet (UV) light is used to manage such situations.

6. Welfare of the Mind and Mood:

- One's mood and mental health can be enhanced by being exposed to natural light. It is believed that being outside and having access to natural light are good for mental health.

7. Awakening with a Blue Light:

- Increased alertness and better cognitive performance have been linked to blue light, particularly when exposed first thing in the morning. This is why some people find that blue-enriched light helps them stay awake during the day.

8. Controlling the Production of Melatonin:

- The hormone melatonin is essential for maintaining regular sleep-wake cycles, and being exposed to light during the day helps control its production.

Although these points show that light has some good benefits, we should be wary of claims that it can cure illnesses. There is less consensus among scientists on chromotherapy, the use of certain colors for medicinal purposes.

Additional research is necessary to gain a comprehensive understanding of the mechanics and effectiveness of chromotherapy, and there is no universal agreement regarding the effects of certain hues on health and wellbeing. Advice based on evidence is best obtained from healthcare experts, as is the case with any health-related activity.

CHAPTER FOUR
Psychology And Chromotherapy

Because colors are recognized to have psychological impacts on our mood, feelings, and behavior, chromotherapy (also called color therapy) is occasionally investigated within the field of psychology.

Color psychology is an established discipline that investigates how different hues influence people's thoughts, feelings, and actions; nevertheless, there is little evidence to support chromotherapy as a separate therapeutic technique.

Some areas where chromotherapy and psychology meet are as follows:

1. The Psychology of Color:

- Color psychology delves at the ways in which different hues might impact our mental states, actions, and emotions. It's a well-established subfield in psychology.

- Colors are thought to have the power to elicit particular feelings in people. For instance, it is commonly believed that warm colors, such as red and orange, evoke feelings of energy and enthusiasm, whilst cool colors, such as blue and green, are linked to feelings of tranquility and rest.

2. Impact on the Environment:

- One common method of chromotherapy is the use of carefully orchestrated color schemes to affect patients' mental health.

- Spaces intended for relaxation might make use of soothing colors like blue or green, while places meant to inspire energy and creativity might make use of bold colors.

3. Elevating Mood:

- According to those who advocate for chromotherapy, being exposed to specific hues can have a favorable effect on one's mood and emotional health.

- As an example, the color yellow is commonly thought of as energetic and positive, but the color blue is typically thought of as calming and serene.

4. Neuro-Endocrine Link:

- The mind-body link is a larger framework within which chromotherapy is occasionally examined. The basic premise is that one can influence one's physiological responses by modifying one's mental perception of color.

5. Chakra Connections:

- Colors are thought to correspond to various energy centers, or chakras, in the body according to several alternative and spiritual healing traditions. It is possible to activate or balance these energy centers with chromotherapy.

6. The Use of Color in the Field of Design Therapy:

- The psychological impacts of color are frequently included into art therapy and interior design. Attractive and comforting spaces can be designed using chromotherapy concepts.

7. Methods for Visualization:

- One form of chromotherapy is visualizing oneself in a certain frame of mind by focusing on or imagining a certain color.

- The scientific community views chromotherapy as a complementary or alternative therapy, and its effectiveness has not been extensively proven via rigorous scientific investigations, but there is anecdotal evidence that colors can impact emotions and well-being.

Different people have different reactions to different colors, and cultural, personal, and environmental factors all play a role in how colors make us feel. It may be subjective and individual if people report feeling better after being among particular hues.

It is important to engage with healthcare specialists for evidence-based recommendations on mental health and well-being, and to pursue chromotherapy with a knowledge of its speculative character.

Chromatography In Context

Some people opt to include color considerations into their daily life for aesthetic or health reasons, even though chromotherapy is not generally acknowledged in mainstream medicine. Here are a few examples of practical applications of chromotherapy principles:

1. Décor for the Home:

- Placing one's own tastes or intended psychological effects as the guiding principles for selecting one's home's paint, furniture, and décor colors.

- Placing soothing hues like greens or blues in bedrooms and other places meant for relaxation and energetic hues like yellows or reds in locations meant for socializing are two examples.

2. Modest Garments and Extras:

- Choosing an outfit and accessories that complement the energy level or mood you want to achieve that day.

- People's psychological associations with particular hues may impact their choice to wear specific colors.

3. Places of Employment:

- Altering the color palette of work areas to promote concentration, inspiration, or calmness.

- For instance, in places that require focus and concentration, calming hues are used, whereas in creative settings, lively colors are used.

4. Options for Lighting:

- Setting the mood in various rooms with the use of colorful light bulbs or programmable LED lights.

- Users can personalize their lighting experience by adjusting the brightness and color temperature of certain smart lighting systems.

5. Arts & Creative Activities:

- Creating works of art or partaking in other creative pursuits that call for the selection of hues to elicit feeling or mood.

6. How to Express Oneself through Clothes:

- Color-coordinating one's wardrobe according to one's own taste or the effect one hopes to achieve at a given event.

- Some people think that certain colors make them feel more confident or energetic.

7. Spending Time in Nature and Gardening:

- Doing things like tending gardens or going for walks in nature while paying attention to the hues of various plants and flowers.

- Paying attention to how different hues in nature affect our emotions and sense of well-being.

8. Visualization and Mindfulness:

- Adding color visualization exercises to mindfulness techniques for use during meditation or relaxation.

- To foster a feeling of calm or happiness, some mindfulness techniques incorporate color imagery.

The precise claims of chromotherapy regarding healing or treating medical conditions lack substantial scientific evidence, while incorporating color preferences into everyday life is a personal choice and may add to a happy environment. Cultural, individual, and environmental variables all have a role in shaping how people perceive and react to color.

Color awareness can be a meaningful and individual kind of self-care if people discover that it improves their mood or overall health. However, it's recommended to seek advice from healthcare professionals who can handle specific health concerns based on evidence.

Summary

Chromotherapy, often called color therapy, is a form of supplementary medicine that proposes the use of specific colors to improve mental and physical health. The psychological effects of color have long been acknowledged, particularly in the domains of color psychology and design. However, chromotherapy's particular assertions and uses have not been well supported by scientific research.

Certain medical settings acknowledge and exploit light's therapeutic power in more established contexts, such as light therapy for wound healing and Seasonal Affective Disorder. Chromatography proposes the use of certain colors for medicinal purposes, however this idea is still controversial and not well-accepted in conventional medicine.

On a daily basis, people's environments, wardrobe choices, and creative expressions can all be influenced by color theory, which is rooted in subjective experiences and the associations people have with specific hues.

Although this can help create a more pleasant and visually attractive atmosphere, one must approach chromotherapy with skepticism and recognize that it is theoretical.

Healthcare providers can offer evidence-based advice and make sure that a person's chosen practices are in line with their overall health and wellness if they consult with them before adopting chromotherapy for health-related reasons. Everyone reacts differently to chromotherapy; therefore, it is important to go into the practice with an open mind, acknowledging that it is subjective, as is the case with many alternative therapies.

THE END